this book
belongs to:

____

____

____

TRACK YOUR PROGRESS

WEIGHT week/month

TRACK:

TRACK:

TRACK:

TRACK:

TRACK:

TRACK:

TRACK YOUR PROGRESS

TRACK:

TRACK:

TRACK:

TRACK:

TRACK:

TRACK:

TRACK:

GOALS

GOALS

Date: ___ / ___ / ___

WHY AM I WORKING OUT TODAY?

So whether you eat or drink or whatever you do, do it all for the glory of God.
1 Corinthians 10:31

TODAY'S WORKOUT GOALS:

EXERCISE	WT/Reps	WT/Reps	WT/Reps	WT/Reps	WT/Reps

CARDIO

EXERCISE	TIME	DISTANCE	REST

WHAT CHALLENGES DID YOU FACE TODAY?

HOW WILL YOU OVERCOME THESE CHALLENGES?

NOTES / PRAYERS / GRATITUDE

WHY AM I WORKING OUT TODAY?

In the same way, let your light shine before others, that they may see your good deeds
and glorify your Father in heaven.
Matthew 5:16

TODAY'S WORKOUT GOALS:

EXERCISE	WT/Reps	WT/Reps	WT/Reps	WT/Reps	WT/Reps

CARDIO

EXERCISE	TIME	DISTANCE	REST

WHAT CHALLENGES DID YOU FACE TODAY?

HOW WILL YOU OVERCOME THESE CHALLENGES?

NOTES / PRAYERS / GRATITUDE

Date: ___ / ___ / ___

WHY AM I WORKING OUT TODAY?

Just as a body, though one, has many parts, but all its many parts form one body, so it is
with Christ.
1 Corinthians 12:12

TODAY'S WORKOUT GOALS:

EXERCISE

EXERCISE	WT/Reps	WT/Reps	WT/Reps	WT/Reps	WT/Reps

CARDIO

EXERCISE	TIME	DISTANCE	REST

WHAT CHALLENGES DID YOU FACE TODAY?

HOW WILL YOU OVERCOME THESE CHALLENGES?

NOTES / PRAYERS / GRATITUDE

Date: ___ / ___ / ___

WHY AM I WORKING OUT TODAY?

Each of you should use whatever gift you have received to serve others, as faithful stewards of God's grace in its various forms.
1 Peter 4:10

TODAY'S WORKOUT GOALS:

EXERCISE	WT/Reps	WT/Reps	WT/Reps	WT/Reps	WT/Reps

CARDIO

EXERCISE	TIME	DISTANCE	REST

WHAT CHALLENGES DID YOU FACE TODAY?

HOW WILL YOU OVERCOME THESE CHALLENGES?

NOTES / PRAYERS / GRATITUDE

Date: ___ / ___ / ___

WHY AM I WORKING OUT TODAY?

____

____

____

____

Whatever you do, work at it with all your heart, as working for the Lord, not for human masters.
Colossians 3:23

TODAY'S WORKOUT GOALS:

____

____

____

____

EXERCISE

	WT/Reps	WT/Reps	WT/Reps	WT/Reps	WT/Reps

CARDIO

EXERCISE	TIME	DISTANCE	REST

WHAT CHALLENGES DID YOU FACE TODAY?

HOW WILL YOU OVERCOME THESE CHALLENGES?

NOTES / PRAYERS / GRATITUDE

Date: ___ / ___ / ___

WHY AM I WORKING OUT TODAY?

Not only so, but we also glory in our sufferings, because we know that suffering produces
perseverance; perseverance, character; and character, hope.
Romans 5:3-4

TODAY'S WORKOUT GOALS:

EXERCISE	WT/Reps	WT/Reps	WT/Reps	WT/Reps	WT/Reps

CARDIO

EXERCISE	TIME	DISTANCE	REST

WHAT CHALLENGES DID YOU FACE TODAY?

HOW WILL YOU OVERCOME THESE CHALLENGES?

NOTES / PRAYERS / GRATITUDE

WHY AM I WORKING OUT TODAY?

Blessed is the one who perseveres under trial because, having stood the test, that person will receive the crown of life that the Lord has promised to those who love him.
James 1:12

TODAY'S WORKOUT GOALS:

EXERCISE

EXERCISE	WT/Reps	WT/Reps	WT/Reps	WT/Reps	WT/Reps

CARDIO

EXERCISE	TIME	DISTANCE	REST

WHAT CHALLENGES DID YOU FACE TODAY?

HOW WILL YOU OVERCOME THESE CHALLENGES?

NOTES / PRAYERS / GRATITUDE

Date: ___ / ___ / ___

WHY AM I WORKING OUT TODAY?

____

____

____

____

Therefore, since we are surrounded by such a great cloud of witnesses, let us throw off everything that hinders and the sin that so easily entangles, and let us run with perseverance the race marked out for us.
Hebrews 12:1

TODAY'S WORKOUT GOALS:

____

____

____

____

EXERCISE

EXERCISE	WT/Reps	WT/Reps	WT/Reps	WT/Reps	WT/Reps

CARDIO

EXERCISE	TIME	DISTANCE	REST

WHAT CHALLENGES DID YOU FACE TODAY?

HOW WILL YOU OVERCOME THESE CHALLENGES?

NOTES / PRAYERS / GRATITUDE

Date: ___ / ___ / ___

WHY AM I WORKING OUT TODAY?

____

____

____

____

> An athlete is not crowned unless he competes according to the rules.
> 2 Timothy 2:5

TODAY'S WORKOUT GOALS:

____

____

____

____

EXERCISE	WT/Reps	WT/Reps	WT/Reps	WT/Reps	WT/Reps

CARDIO

EXERCISE	TIME	DISTANCE	REST

WHAT CHALLENGES DID YOU FACE TODAY?

HOW WILL YOU OVERCOME THESE CHALLENGES?

NOTES / PRAYERS / GRATITUDE

Date: ___ / ___ / ___

WHY AM I WORKING OUT TODAY?

A man without self-control is like a city broken into and left without walls.
Proverbs 25:28

TODAY'S WORKOUT GOALS:

EXERCISE	WT/Reps	WT/Reps	WT/Reps	WT/Reps	WT/Reps

CARDIO

EXERCISE	TIME	DISTANCE	REST

WHAT CHALLENGES DID YOU FACE TODAY?

HOW WILL YOU OVERCOME THESE CHALLENGES?

NOTES / PRAYERS / GRATITUDE

WHY AM I WORKING OUT TODAY?

But the fruit of the Spirit is love, joy, peace, patience, kindness, goodness, faithfulness, gentleness, and self-control. Against such things, there is no law.
Galatians 5:22-23

TODAY'S WORKOUT GOALS:

EXERCISE	WT/Reps	WT/Reps	WT/Reps	WT/Reps	WT/Reps

CARDIO

EXERCISE	TIME	DISTANCE	REST

WHAT CHALLENGES DID YOU FACE TODAY?

HOW WILL YOU OVERCOME THESE CHALLENGES?

NOTES / PRAYERS / GRATITUDE

Date: ___ / ___ / ___

WHY AM I WORKING OUT TODAY?

Do you not know that in a race all the runners run, but only one gets the prize? Run in such a way as to get the prize.
1 Corinthians 9:24-27

TODAY'S WORKOUT GOALS:

EXERCISE	WT/Reps	WT/Reps	WT/Reps	WT/Reps	WT/Reps

CARDIO

EXERCISE	TIME	DISTANCE	REST

WHAT CHALLENGES DID YOU FACE TODAY?

HOW WILL YOU OVERCOME THESE CHALLENGES?

NOTES / PRAYERS / GRATITUDE

Date: ___ / ___ / ___

WHY AM I WORKING OUT TODAY?

Finally, be strong in the Lord and in his mighty power.
Ephesians 6:10

TODAY'S WORKOUT GOALS:

EXERCISE	WT/Reps	WT/Reps	WT/Reps	WT/Reps	WT/Reps

CARDIO

EXERCISE	TIME	DISTANCE	REST

WHAT CHALLENGES DID YOU FACE TODAY?

HOW WILL YOU OVERCOME THESE CHALLENGES?

NOTES / PRAYERS / GRATITUDE

Date: ___ / ___ / ___

WHY AM I WORKING OUT TODAY?

For God has not given us a spirit of fear, but of power and of love and of a sound mind.
2 Timothy 1:7

TODAY'S WORKOUT GOALS:

EXERCISE

	WT/Reps	WT/Reps	WT/Reps	WT/Reps	WT/Reps

CARDIO

EXERCISE	TIME	DISTANCE	REST

WHAT CHALLENGES DID YOU FACE TODAY?

HOW WILL YOU OVERCOME THESE CHALLENGES?

NOTES / PRAYERS / GRATITUDE

Date: ___ / ___ / ___

WHY AM I WORKING OUT TODAY?

Be on your guard; stand firm in the faith; be courageous; be strong.
1 Corinthians 16:13

TODAY'S WORKOUT GOALS:

EXERCISE	WT/Reps	WT/Reps	WT/Reps	WT/Reps	WT/Reps

CARDIO

EXERCISE	TIME	DISTANCE	REST

WHAT CHALLENGES DID YOU FACE TODAY?

HOW WILL YOU OVERCOME THESE CHALLENGES?

NOTES / PRAYERS / GRATITUDE

Date: ___ / ___ / ___

WHY AM I WORKING OUT TODAY?

> But those who hope in the Lord will renew their strength. They will soar on wings like eagles; they will run and not grow weary, they will walk and not be faint.
> Isaiah 40:31

TODAY'S WORKOUT GOALS:

EXERCISE	WT/Reps	WT/Reps	WT/Reps	WT/Reps	WT/Reps

CARDIO

EXERCISE	TIME	DISTANCE	REST

WHAT CHALLENGES DID YOU FACE TODAY?

HOW WILL YOU OVERCOME THESE CHALLENGES?

NOTES / PRAYERS / GRATITUDE

WHY AM I WORKING OUT TODAY?

So whether you eat or drink or whatever you do, do it all for the glory of God.
1 Corinthians 10:31

TODAY'S WORKOUT GOALS:

EXERCISE	WT / Reps	WT / Reps	WT / Reps	WT / Reps	WT / Reps

CARDIO

EXERCISE	TIME	DISTANCE	REST

WHAT CHALLENGES DID YOU FACE TODAY?

HOW WILL YOU OVERCOME THESE CHALLENGES?

NOTES / PRAYERS / GRATITUDE

WHY AM I WORKING OUT TODAY?

In the same way, let your light shine before others, that they may see your good deeds
and glorify your Father in heaven.
Matthew 5:16

TODAY'S WORKOUT GOALS:

EXERCISE	WT/Reps	WT/Reps	WT/Reps	WT/Reps	WT/Reps

CARDIO

EXERCISE	TIME	DISTANCE	REST

WHAT CHALLENGES DID YOU FACE TODAY?

HOW WILL YOU OVERCOME THESE CHALLENGES?

NOTES / PRAYERS / GRATITUDE

Date: ___ / ___ / ___

WHY AM I WORKING OUT TODAY?

Just as a body, though one, has many parts, but all its many parts form one body, so it is
with Christ.
1 Corinthians 12:12

TODAY'S WORKOUT GOALS:

EXERCISE	WT/Reps	WT/Reps	WT/Reps	WT/Reps	WT/Reps

CARDIO

EXERCISE	TIME	DISTANCE	REST

WHAT CHALLENGES DID YOU FACE TODAY?

HOW WILL YOU OVERCOME THESE CHALLENGES?

NOTES / PRAYERS / GRATITUDE

WHY AM I WORKING OUT TODAY?

Or do you not know that your body is a temple of the Holy Spirit within you, whom you have from God? You are not your own, for you were bought with a price. So glorify God in your body.
1 Corinthians 6:19-20

TODAY'S WORKOUT GOALS:

EXERCISE	WT/Reps	WT/Reps	WT/Reps	WT/Reps	WT/Reps

CARDIO

EXERCISE	TIME	DISTANCE	REST

WHAT CHALLENGES DID YOU FACE TODAY?

HOW WILL YOU OVERCOME THESE CHALLENGES?

NOTES / PRAYERS / GRATITUDE

Date: ___ / ___ / ___

WHY AM I WORKING OUT TODAY?

But I discipline my body and keep it under control, lest after preaching to others I myself
should be disqualified.
1 Corinthians 9:27

TODAY'S WORKOUT GOALS:

EXERCISE	WT/Reps	WT/Reps	WT/Reps	WT/Reps	WT/Reps

CARDIO

EXERCISE	TIME	DISTANCE	REST

WHAT CHALLENGES DID YOU FACE TODAY?

HOW WILL YOU OVERCOME THESE CHALLENGES?

NOTES / PRAYERS / GRATITUDE

Date: ___ / ___ / ___

WHY AM I WORKING OUT TODAY?

So whether you eat or drink or whatever you do, do it all for the glory of God.
1 Corinthians 10:31

TODAY'S WORKOUT GOALS:

EXERCISE	WT/Reps	WT/Reps	WT/Reps	WT/Reps	WT/Reps

CARDIO

EXERCISE	TIME	DISTANCE	REST

WHAT CHALLENGES DID YOU FACE TODAY?

HOW WILL YOU OVERCOME THESE CHALLENGES?

NOTES / PRAYERS / GRATITUDE

Date: ___ / ___ / ___

WHY AM I WORKING OUT TODAY?

Each one should test his own actions. Then he can take pride in himself, without comparing himself to somebody else.
Galatians 6:4

TODAY'S WORKOUT GOALS:

EXERCISE	WT/Reps	WT/Reps	WT/Reps	WT/Reps	WT/Reps

CARDIO

EXERCISE	TIME	DISTANCE	REST

WHAT CHALLENGES DID YOU FACE TODAY?

HOW WILL YOU OVERCOME THESE CHALLENGES?

NOTES / PRAYERS / GRATITUDE

Date: ___ / ___ / ___

WHY AM I WORKING OUT TODAY?

Therefore take up the whole armor of God, that you may be able to withstand in the evil day, and having done all, to stand firm.
Ephesians 6:13

TODAY'S WORKOUT GOALS:

EXERCISE	WT/Reps	WT/Reps	WT/Reps	WT/Reps	WT/Reps

CARDIO

EXERCISE	TIME	DISTANCE	REST

WHAT CHALLENGES DID YOU FACE TODAY?

HOW WILL YOU OVERCOME THESE CHALLENGES?

NOTES / PRAYERS / GRATITUDE

WHY AM I WORKING OUT TODAY?

Each of you should use whatever gift you have received to serve others, as faithful
stewards of God's grace in its various forms.
1 Peter 4:10

TODAY'S WORKOUT GOALS:

EXERCISE	WT/Reps	WT/Reps	WT/Reps	WT/Reps	WT/Reps

CARDIO

EXERCISE	TIME	DISTANCE	REST

WHAT CHALLENGES DID YOU FACE TODAY?

HOW WILL YOU OVERCOME THESE CHALLENGES?

NOTES / PRAYERS / GRATITUDE

WHY AM I WORKING OUT TODAY?

Whatever you do, work at it with all your heart, as working for the Lord, not for human masters.
Colossians 3:23

TODAY'S WORKOUT GOALS:

EXERCISE

	WT/Reps	WT/Reps	WT/Reps	WT/Reps	WT/Reps

CARDIO

EXERCISE	TIME	DISTANCE	REST

WHAT CHALLENGES DID YOU FACE TODAY?

HOW WILL YOU OVERCOME THESE CHALLENGES?

NOTES / PRAYERS / GRATITUDE

WHY AM I WORKING OUT TODAY?

But the Lord said to Samuel, Do not look on his appearance or on the height of his stature, because I have rejected him. For the Lord sees not as man sees: man looks on the outward appearance, but the Lord looks on the heart.
1 Samuel 16:7

TODAY'S WORKOUT GOALS:

EXERCISE	WT/Reps	WT/Reps	WT/Reps	WT/Reps	WT/Reps

CARDIO

EXERCISE	TIME	DISTANCE	REST

WHAT CHALLENGES DID YOU FACE TODAY?

HOW WILL YOU OVERCOME THESE CHALLENGES?

NOTES / PRAYERS / GRATITUDE

WHY AM I WORKING OUT TODAY?

Commit your way to the LORD; trust in him, and he will act.
Psalm 37:5

TODAY'S WORKOUT GOALS:

EXERCISE

EXERCISE	WT/Reps	WT/Reps	WT/Reps	WT/Reps	WT/Reps

CARDIO

EXERCISE	TIME	DISTANCE	REST

WHAT CHALLENGES DID YOU FACE TODAY?

HOW WILL YOU OVERCOME THESE CHALLENGES?

NOTES / PRAYERS / GRATITUDE

WHY AM I WORKING OUT TODAY?

____

____

____

____

The steps of a man are established by the LORD, when he delights in his way though he
fall, he shall not be cast headlong, for the LORD upholds his hand.
Psalm 37:23-24

TODAY'S WORKOUT GOALS:

____

____

____

____

EXERCISE	WT/Reps	WT/Reps	WT/Reps	WT/Reps	WT/Reps

CARDIO

EXERCISE	TIME	DISTANCE	REST

WHAT CHALLENGES DID YOU FACE TODAY?

HOW WILL YOU OVERCOME THESE CHALLENGES?

NOTES / PRAYERS / GRATITUDE

Date: ___ / ___ / ___

WHY AM I WORKING OUT TODAY?

The road to life is a disciplined life; ignore correction and you're lost for good.
Proverbs 10:17

TODAY'S WORKOUT GOALS:

EXERCISE	WT/Reps	WT/Reps	WT/Reps	WT/Reps	WT/Reps

CARDIO

EXERCISE	TIME	DISTANCE	REST

WHAT CHALLENGES DID YOU FACE TODAY?

HOW WILL YOU OVERCOME THESE CHALLENGES?

NOTES / PRAYERS / GRATITUDE

WHY AM I WORKING OUT TODAY?

He who works his land will have abundant food, but he who chases fantasies lacks judgment.
Proverbs 12:11

TODAY'S WORKOUT GOALS:

EXERCISE	WT/Reps	WT/Reps	WT/Reps	WT/Reps	WT/Reps

CARDIO

EXERCISE	TIME	DISTANCE	REST

WHAT CHALLENGES DID YOU FACE TODAY?

HOW WILL YOU OVERCOME THESE CHALLENGES?

NOTES / PRAYERS / GRATITUDE

WHY AM I WORKING OUT TODAY?

____

____

____

____

For while bodily training is of some value, godliness is of value in every way, as it holds promise for the present life and also for the life to come.
1 Timothy 4:8

TODAY'S WORKOUT GOALS:

____

____

____

____

EXERCISE	WT / Reps	WT / Reps	WT / Reps	WT / Reps	WT / Reps

CARDIO

EXERCISE	TIME	DISTANCE	REST

WHAT CHALLENGES DID YOU FACE TODAY?

HOW WILL YOU OVERCOME THESE CHALLENGES?

NOTES / PRAYERS / GRATITUDE

Date: ___ / ___ / ___

WHY AM I WORKING OUT TODAY?

I have fought the good fight, I have finished the race, I have kept the faith.
2 Timothy 4:7

TODAY'S WORKOUT GOALS:

EXERCISE	WT/Reps	WT/Reps	WT/Reps	WT/Reps	WT/Reps

CARDIO

EXERCISE	TIME	DISTANCE	REST

WHAT CHALLENGES DID YOU FACE TODAY?

HOW WILL YOU OVERCOME THESE CHALLENGES?

NOTES / PRAYERS / GRATITUDE

WHY AM I WORKING OUT TODAY?

____

____

____

____

For the moment all discipline seems painful rather than pleasant, but later it yields the
peaceful fruit of righteousness to those who have been trained by it.
Hebrews 12:11

TODAY'S WORKOUT GOALS:

____

____

____

____

EXERCISE	WT/Reps	WT/Reps	WT/Reps	WT/Reps	WT/Reps

CARDIO

EXERCISE	TIME	DISTANCE	REST

WHAT CHALLENGES DID YOU FACE TODAY?

HOW WILL YOU OVERCOME THESE CHALLENGES?

NOTES / PRAYERS / GRATITUDE

Date: ___ / ___ / ___

WHY AM I WORKING OUT TODAY?

Beloved, I pray that all may go well with you and that you may be in good health, as it goes well with your soul.
3 John 1:2

TODAY'S WORKOUT GOALS:

EXERCISE	WT/Reps	WT/Reps	WT/Reps	WT/Reps	WT/Reps

CARDIO

EXERCISE	TIME	DISTANCE	REST

WHAT CHALLENGES DID YOU FACE TODAY?

HOW WILL YOU OVERCOME THESE CHALLENGES?

NOTES / PRAYERS / GRATITUDE

WHY AM I WORKING OUT TODAY?

Behold, I am coming soon, bringing my recompense with me, to repay everyone for what he has done. I am the Alpha and the Omega, the first and the last, the beginning and the end.
Revelation 22:12-13

TODAY'S WORKOUT GOALS:

EXERCISE	WT/Reps	WT/Reps	WT/Reps	WT/Reps	WT/Reps

CARDIO

EXERCISE	TIME	DISTANCE	REST

WHAT CHALLENGES DID YOU FACE TODAY?

HOW WILL YOU OVERCOME THESE CHALLENGES?

NOTES / PRAYERS / GRATITUDE

WHY AM I WORKING OUT TODAY?

All hard work brings a profit, but mere talk leads only to poverty.
Proverbs 14:23

TODAY'S WORKOUT GOALS:

EXERCISE	WT/Reps	WT/Reps	WT/Reps	WT/Reps	WT/Reps

CARDIO

EXERCISE	TIME	DISTANCE	REST

WHAT CHALLENGES DID YOU FACE TODAY?

HOW WILL YOU OVERCOME THESE CHALLENGES?

NOTES / PRAYERS / GRATITUDE

Date: ___ / ___ / ___

WHY AM I WORKING OUT TODAY?

She dresses herself with strength and makes her arms strong.
Proverbs 31:17

TODAY'S WORKOUT GOALS:

EXERCISE

EXERCISE	WT/Reps	WT/Reps	WT/Reps	WT/Reps	WT/Reps

CARDIO

EXERCISE	TIME	DISTANCE	REST

WHAT CHALLENGES DID YOU FACE TODAY?

HOW WILL YOU OVERCOME THESE CHALLENGES?

NOTES / PRAYERS / GRATITUDE

WHY AM I WORKING OUT TODAY?

Strength and dignity are her clothing, and she smiles at the future.
Proverbs 31:25

TODAY'S WORKOUT GOALS:

EXERCISE	WT/Reps	WT/Reps	WT/Reps	WT/Reps	WT/Reps

CARDIO

EXERCISE	TIME	DISTANCE	REST

WHAT CHALLENGES DID YOU FACE TODAY?

HOW WILL YOU OVERCOME THESE CHALLENGES?

NOTES / PRAYERS / GRATITUDE

Date: ___ / ___ / ___

WHY AM I WORKING OUT TODAY?

Though one may be overpowered, two can defend themselves. A cord of three strands is not quickly broken.
Ecclesiastes 4:12

TODAY'S WORKOUT GOALS:

EXERCISE	WT/Reps	WT/Reps	WT/Reps	WT/Reps	WT/Reps

CARDIO

EXERCISE	TIME	DISTANCE	REST

WHAT CHALLENGES DID YOU FACE TODAY?

HOW WILL YOU OVERCOME THESE CHALLENGES?

NOTES / PRAYERS / GRATITUDE

WHY AM I WORKING OUT TODAY?

> The LORD will guide you continually, watering your life when you are dry and keeping you healthy, too. You will be like a well-watered garden, like an ever-flowing spring.
> Isaiah 58:11

TODAY'S WORKOUT GOALS:

EXERCISE	WT/Reps	WT/Reps	WT/Reps	WT/Reps	WT/Reps

CARDIO

EXERCISE	TIME	DISTANCE	REST

WHAT CHALLENGES DID YOU FACE TODAY?

HOW WILL YOU OVERCOME THESE CHALLENGES?

NOTES / PRAYERS / GRATITUDE

Date: ___ / ___ / ___

WHY AM I WORKING OUT TODAY?

People need more than bread for their life; they must feed on every word of God.
Matthew 4:4

TODAY'S WORKOUT GOALS:

EXERCISE	WT/Reps	WT/Reps	WT/Reps	WT/Reps	WT/Reps

CARDIO

EXERCISE	TIME	DISTANCE	REST

WHAT CHALLENGES DID YOU FACE TODAY?

HOW WILL YOU OVERCOME THESE CHALLENGES?

NOTES / PRAYERS / GRATITUDE

WHY AM I WORKING OUT TODAY?

You're blessed when you've worked up a good appetite for God. He's food and drink in the best meal you'll ever eat.
Matthew 5:6

TODAY'S WORKOUT GOALS:

EXERCISE

	WT/Reps	WT/Reps	WT/Reps	WT/Reps	WT/Reps

CARDIO

EXERCISE	TIME	DISTANCE	REST

WHAT CHALLENGES DID YOU FACE TODAY?

HOW WILL YOU OVERCOME THESE CHALLENGES?

NOTES / PRAYERS / GRATITUDE

WHY AM I WORKING OUT TODAY?

But Jesus looked at them and said, "With man this is impossible, but with God all things are possible.
Matthew 19:26

TODAY'S WORKOUT GOALS:

EXERCISE

EXERCISE	WT/Reps	WT/Reps	WT/Reps	WT/Reps	WT/Reps

CARDIO

EXERCISE	TIME	DISTANCE	REST

WHAT CHALLENGES DID YOU FACE TODAY?

HOW WILL YOU OVERCOME THESE CHALLENGES?

NOTES / PRAYERS / GRATITUDE

WHY AM I WORKING OUT TODAY?

____

____

____

____

I appeal to you therefore, brothers, by the mercies of God, to present your bodies as a living sacrifice, holy and acceptable to God, which is your spiritual worship.
Romans 12:1

TODAY'S WORKOUT GOALS:

____

____

____

____

EXERCISE	WT/Reps	WT/Reps	WT/Reps	WT/Reps	WT/Reps

CARDIO

EXERCISE	TIME	DISTANCE	REST

WHAT CHALLENGES DID YOU FACE TODAY?

HOW WILL YOU OVERCOME THESE CHALLENGES?

NOTES / PRAYERS / GRATITUDE

Date: ___ / ___ / ___

WHY AM I WORKING OUT TODAY?

Or do you not know that your body is a temple of the Holy Spirit within you, whom you have from God? You are not your own, for you were bought with a price. So glorify God in your body.
1 Corinthians 6:19-20

TODAY'S WORKOUT GOALS:

EXERCISE	WT/Reps	WT/Reps	WT/Reps	WT/Reps	WT/Reps

CARDIO

EXERCISE	TIME	DISTANCE	REST

WHAT CHALLENGES DID YOU FACE TODAY?

HOW WILL YOU OVERCOME THESE CHALLENGES?

NOTES / PRAYERS / GRATITUDE

Date: ___ / ___ / ___

WHY AM I WORKING OUT TODAY?

I pray that out of his glorious riches he may strengthen you with power through his Spirit in your inner being, so that Christ may dwell in your hearts through faith. And I pray that you, being rooted and established in love.
Ephesians 3:16-17

TODAY'S WORKOUT GOALS:

EXERCISE

EXERCISE	WT/Reps	WT/Reps	WT/Reps	WT/Reps	WT/Reps

CARDIO

EXERCISE	TIME	DISTANCE	REST

WHAT CHALLENGES DID YOU FACE TODAY?

HOW WILL YOU OVERCOME THESE CHALLENGES?

NOTES / PRAYERS / GRATITUDE

Date: ___ / ___ / ___

WHY AM I WORKING OUT TODAY?

Now faith is confidence in what we hope for and assurance about what we do not see.
Hebrews 11:1

TODAY'S WORKOUT GOALS:

EXERCISE	WT/Reps	WT/Reps	WT/Reps	WT/Reps	WT/Reps

CARDIO

EXERCISE	TIME	DISTANCE	REST

WHAT CHALLENGES DID YOU FACE TODAY?

HOW WILL YOU OVERCOME THESE CHALLENGES?

NOTES / PRAYERS / GRATITUDE

Date: ___ / ___ / ___

WHY AM I WORKING OUT TODAY?

For we live by faith, not by sight.
2 Corinthians 5:7

TODAY'S WORKOUT GOALS:

EXERCISE	WT/Reps	WT/Reps	WT/Reps	WT/Reps	WT/Reps

CARDIO

EXERCISE	TIME	DISTANCE	REST

WHAT CHALLENGES DID YOU FACE TODAY?

HOW WILL YOU OVERCOME THESE CHALLENGES?

NOTES / PRAYERS / GRATITUDE

Date: ___ / ___ / ___

WHY AM I WORKING OUT TODAY?

May the God of hope fill you with all joy and peace as you trust in him, so that you may
overflow with hope by the power of the Holy Spirit.
Romans 15:13

TODAY'S WORKOUT GOALS:

EXERCISE	WT/Reps	WT/Reps	WT/Reps	WT/Reps	WT/Reps

CARDIO

EXERCISE	TIME	DISTANCE	REST

WHAT CHALLENGES DID YOU FACE TODAY?

HOW WILL YOU OVERCOME THESE CHALLENGES?

NOTES / PRAYERS / GRATITUDE

WHY AM I WORKING OUT TODAY?

But when you ask, you must believe and not doubt, because the one who doubts is like a wave of the sea, blown and tossed by the wind.
James 1:6

TODAY'S WORKOUT GOALS:

EXERCISE	WT/Reps	WT/Reps	WT/Reps	WT/Reps	WT/Reps

CARDIO

EXERCISE	TIME	DISTANCE	REST

WHAT CHALLENGES DID YOU FACE TODAY?

HOW WILL YOU OVERCOME THESE CHALLENGES?

NOTES / PRAYERS / GRATITUDE

WHY AM I WORKING OUT TODAY?

But I discipline my body and keep it under control, lest after preaching to others I myself
should be disqualified.
1 Corinthians 9:27

TODAY'S WORKOUT GOALS:

EXERCISE	WT/Reps	WT/Reps	WT/Reps	WT/Reps	WT/Reps

CARDIO

EXERCISE	TIME	DISTANCE	REST

WHAT CHALLENGES DID YOU FACE TODAY?

HOW WILL YOU OVERCOME THESE CHALLENGES?

NOTES / PRAYERS / GRATITUDE

Date: ___ / ___ / ___

WHY AM I WORKING OUT TODAY?

So whether you eat or drink or whatever you do, do it all for the glory of God.
1 Corinthians 10:31

TODAY'S WORKOUT GOALS:

EXERCISE	WT/Reps	WT/Reps	WT/Reps	WT/Reps	WT/Reps

CARDIO

EXERCISE	TIME	DISTANCE	REST

WHAT CHALLENGES DID YOU FACE TODAY?

HOW WILL YOU OVERCOME THESE CHALLENGES?

NOTES / PRAYERS / GRATITUDE

WHY AM I WORKING OUT TODAY?

____

____

____

____

Each one should test his own actions. Then he can take pride in himself, without comparing himself to somebody else.
Galatians 6:4

TODAY'S WORKOUT GOALS:

____

____

____

____

EXERCISE	WT/Reps	WT/Reps	WT/Reps	WT/Reps	WT/Reps

CARDIO

EXERCISE	TIME	DISTANCE	REST

WHAT CHALLENGES DID YOU FACE TODAY?

HOW WILL YOU OVERCOME THESE CHALLENGES?

NOTES / PRAYERS / GRATITUDE

WHY AM I WORKING OUT TODAY?

Therefore take up the whole armor of God, that you may be able to withstand in the evil day, and having done all, to stand firm.
Ephesians 6:13

TODAY'S WORKOUT GOALS:

EXERCISE	WT/Reps	WT/Reps	WT/Reps	WT/Reps	WT/Reps

CARDIO

EXERCISE	TIME	DISTANCE	REST

WHAT CHALLENGES DID YOU FACE TODAY?

HOW WILL YOU OVERCOME THESE CHALLENGES?

NOTES / PRAYERS / GRATITUDE

WHY AM I WORKING OUT TODAY?

Don't you know that you yourselves are God's temple and that God's Spirit lives in you?
If anyone destroys God's temple, God will destroy him; for God's temple is sacred, and
you are that temple.
1 Corinthians 3:16-17

TODAY'S WORKOUT GOALS:

EXERCISE

	WT/Reps	WT/Reps	WT/Reps	WT/Reps	WT/Reps

CARDIO

EXERCISE	TIME	DISTANCE	REST

WHAT CHALLENGES DID YOU FACE TODAY?

HOW WILL YOU OVERCOME THESE CHALLENGES?

NOTES / PRAYERS / GRATITUDE

WHY AM I WORKING OUT TODAY?

Everything is permissible for me – but not everything is beneficial. Everything is permissible for me – but I will not be mastered by anything.
1 Corinthians 6:12

TODAY'S WORKOUT GOALS:

EXERCISE	WT/Reps	WT/Reps	WT/Reps	WT/Reps	WT/Reps

CARDIO

EXERCISE	TIME	DISTANCE	REST

WHAT CHALLENGES DID YOU FACE TODAY?

HOW WILL YOU OVERCOME THESE CHALLENGES?

NOTES / PRAYERS / GRATITUDE

WHY AM I WORKING OUT TODAY?

Or do you not know that your body is a temple of the Holy Spirit within you, whom you have from God? You are not your own, for you were bought with a price. So glorify God in your body.
1 Corinthians 6:19-20

TODAY'S WORKOUT GOALS:

EXERCISE	WT/Reps	WT/Reps	WT/Reps	WT/Reps	WT/Reps

CARDIO

EXERCISE	TIME	DISTANCE	REST

WHAT CHALLENGES DID YOU FACE TODAY?

HOW WILL YOU OVERCOME THESE CHALLENGES?

NOTES / PRAYERS / GRATITUDE

Date: ___ / ___ / ___

WHY AM I WORKING OUT TODAY?

____

____

____

____

But I discipline my body and keep it under control, lest after preaching to others I myself
should be disqualified.
1 Corinthians 9:27

TODAY'S WORKOUT GOALS:

____

____

____

____

EXERCISE	WT/Reps	WT/Reps	WT/Reps	WT/Reps	WT/Reps

CARDIO

EXERCISE	TIME	DISTANCE	REST

WHAT CHALLENGES DID YOU FACE TODAY?

HOW WILL YOU OVERCOME THESE CHALLENGES?

NOTES / PRAYERS / GRATITUDE

WHY AM I WORKING OUT TODAY?

So whether you eat or drink or whatever you do, do it all for the glory of God.
1 Corinthians 10:31

TODAY'S WORKOUT GOALS:

EXERCISE	WT/Reps	WT/Reps	WT/Reps	WT/Reps	WT/Reps

CARDIO

EXERCISE	TIME	DISTANCE	REST

WHAT CHALLENGES DID YOU FACE TODAY?

HOW WILL YOU OVERCOME THESE CHALLENGES?

NOTES / PRAYERS / GRATITUDE

WHY AM I WORKING OUT TODAY?

> Each one should test his own actions. Then he can take pride in himself, without comparing himself to somebody else.
> Galatians 6:4

TODAY'S WORKOUT GOALS:

EXERCISE	WT/Reps	WT/Reps	WT/Reps	WT/Reps	WT/Reps

CARDIO

EXERCISE	TIME	DISTANCE	REST

WHAT CHALLENGES DID YOU FACE TODAY?

HOW WILL YOU OVERCOME THESE CHALLENGES?

NOTES / PRAYERS / GRATITUDE

Date: ___ / ___ / ___

WHY AM I WORKING OUT TODAY?

Therefore take up the whole armor of God, that you may be able to withstand in the evil day, and having done all, to stand firm.
Ephesians 6:13

TODAY'S WORKOUT GOALS:

EXERCISE	WT/Reps	WT/Reps	WT/Reps	WT/Reps	WT/Reps

CARDIO

EXERCISE	TIME	DISTANCE	REST

WHAT CHALLENGES DID YOU FACE TODAY?

HOW WILL YOU OVERCOME THESE CHALLENGES?

NOTES / PRAYERS / GRATITUDE

WHY AM I WORKING OUT TODAY?

Finally, be strong in the Lord and in his mighty power.
Ephesians 6:10

TODAY'S WORKOUT GOALS:

EXERCISE

EXERCISE	WT/Reps	WT/Reps	WT/Reps	WT/Reps	WT/Reps

CARDIO

EXERCISE	TIME	DISTANCE	REST

WHAT CHALLENGES DID YOU FACE TODAY?

HOW WILL YOU OVERCOME THESE CHALLENGES?

NOTES / PRAYERS / GRATITUDE

WHY AM I WORKING OUT TODAY?

For God has not given us a spirit of fear, but of power and of love and of a sound mind.
2 Timothy 1:7

TODAY'S WORKOUT GOALS:

EXERCISE	WT/Reps	WT/Reps	WT/Reps	WT/Reps	WT/Reps

CARDIO

EXERCISE	TIME	DISTANCE	REST

WHAT CHALLENGES DID YOU FACE TODAY?

HOW WILL YOU OVERCOME THESE CHALLENGES?

NOTES / PRAYERS / GRATITUDE

WHY AM I WORKING OUT TODAY?

Be on your guard; stand firm in the faith; be courageous; be strong.
1 Corinthians 16:13

TODAY'S WORKOUT GOALS:

EXERCISE	WT/Reps	WT/Reps	WT/Reps	WT/Reps	WT/Reps

CARDIO

EXERCISE	TIME	DISTANCE	REST

WHAT CHALLENGES DID YOU FACE TODAY?

HOW WILL YOU OVERCOME THESE CHALLENGES?

NOTES / PRAYERS / GRATITUDE

WHY AM I WORKING OUT TODAY?

But those who hope in the Lord will renew their strength. They will soar on wings like eagles; they will run and not grow weary, they will walk and not be faint.
Isaiah 40:31

TODAY'S WORKOUT GOALS:

EXERCISE	WT/Reps	WT/Reps	WT/Reps	WT/Reps	WT/Reps

CARDIO

EXERCISE	TIME	DISTANCE	REST

WHAT CHALLENGES DID YOU FACE TODAY?

HOW WILL YOU OVERCOME THESE CHALLENGES?

NOTES / PRAYERS / GRATITUDE

Date: ___ / ___ / ___

WHY AM I WORKING OUT TODAY?

So whether you eat or drink or whatever you do, do it all for the glory of God.
1 Corinthians 10:31

TODAY'S WORKOUT GOALS:

EXERCISE	WT/Reps	WT/Reps	WT/Reps	WT/Reps	WT/Reps

CARDIO

EXERCISE	TIME	DISTANCE	REST

WHAT CHALLENGES DID YOU FACE TODAY?

HOW WILL YOU OVERCOME THESE CHALLENGES?

NOTES / PRAYERS / GRATITUDE

WHY AM I WORKING OUT TODAY?

____

____

____

____

Do not be anxious about anything, but in everything, by prayer and petition, with thanksgiving, present your requests to God. And the peace of God, which transcends all understanding, will guard your hearts and your minds in Christ Jesus.
Philippians 4:6-7

TODAY'S WORKOUT GOALS:

____

____

____

____

EXERCISE	WT/Reps	WT/Reps	WT/Reps	WT/Reps	WT/Reps

CARDIO

EXERCISE	TIME	DISTANCE	REST

WHAT CHALLENGES DID YOU FACE TODAY?

HOW WILL YOU OVERCOME THESE CHALLENGES?

NOTES / PRAYERS / GRATITUDE

Date: ___ / ___ / ___

WHY AM I WORKING OUT TODAY?

I can do all things through him who strengthens me.
Philippians 4:13

TODAY'S WORKOUT GOALS:

EXERCISE	WT/Reps	WT/Reps	WT/Reps	WT/Reps	WT/Reps

CARDIO

EXERCISE	TIME	DISTANCE	REST

WHAT CHALLENGES DID YOU FACE TODAY?

HOW WILL YOU OVERCOME THESE CHALLENGES?

NOTES / PRAYERS / GRATITUDE

Date: ___ / ___ / ___

WHY AM I WORKING OUT TODAY?

Brothers and sisters, we urge you to warn those who are lazy. Encourage those who are timid. Take tender care of those who are weak. Be patient with everyone.
1 Thessalonians 5:14

TODAY'S WORKOUT GOALS:

EXERCISE	WT/Reps	WT/Reps	WT/Reps	WT/Reps	WT/Reps

CARDIO

EXERCISE	TIME	DISTANCE	REST

WHAT CHALLENGES DID YOU FACE TODAY?

HOW WILL YOU OVERCOME THESE CHALLENGES?

NOTES / PRAYERS / GRATITUDE

WHY AM I WORKING OUT TODAY?

For even when we were with you, we would give you this command: If anyone is not willing to work, let him not eat.
2 Thessalonians 3:10

TODAY'S WORKOUT GOALS:

EXERCISE

EXERCISE	WT/Reps	WT/Reps	WT/Reps	WT/Reps	WT/Reps

CARDIO

EXERCISE	TIME	DISTANCE	REST

WHAT CHALLENGES DID YOU FACE TODAY?

HOW WILL YOU OVERCOME THESE CHALLENGES?

NOTES / PRAYERS / GRATITUDE

Date: ___ / ___ / ___

WHY AM I WORKING OUT TODAY?

For while bodily training is of some value, godliness is of value in every way, as it holds promise for the present life and also for the life to come.
1 Timothy 4:8

TODAY'S WORKOUT GOALS:

EXERCISE	WT/Reps	WT/Reps	WT/Reps	WT/Reps	WT/Reps

CARDIO

EXERCISE	TIME	DISTANCE	REST

WHAT CHALLENGES DID YOU FACE TODAY?

HOW WILL YOU OVERCOME THESE CHALLENGES?

NOTES / PRAYERS / GRATITUDE

WHY AM I WORKING OUT TODAY?

I have fought the good fight, I have finished the race, I have kept the faith.
2 Timothy 4:7

TODAY'S WORKOUT GOALS:

EXERCISE	WT/Reps	WT/Reps	WT/Reps	WT/Reps	WT/Reps

CARDIO

EXERCISE	TIME	DISTANCE	REST

WHAT CHALLENGES DID YOU FACE TODAY?

HOW WILL YOU OVERCOME THESE CHALLENGES?

NOTES / PRAYERS / GRATITUDE

Date: ___ / ___ / ___

WHY AM I WORKING OUT TODAY?

For the moment all discipline seems painful rather than pleasant, but later it yields the
peaceful fruit of righteousness to those who have been trained by it.
Hebrews 12:11

TODAY'S WORKOUT GOALS:

EXERCISE	WT/Reps	WT/Reps	WT/Reps	WT/Reps	WT/Reps

CARDIO

EXERCISE	TIME	DISTANCE	REST

WHAT CHALLENGES DID YOU FACE TODAY?

HOW WILL YOU OVERCOME THESE CHALLENGES?

NOTES / PRAYERS / GRATITUDE

WHY AM I WORKING OUT TODAY?

> Beloved, I pray that all may go well with you and that you may be in good health, as it goes well with your soul.
> 3 John 1:2

TODAY'S WORKOUT GOALS:

EXERCISE

EXERCISE	WT/Reps	WT/Reps	WT/Reps	WT/Reps	WT/Reps

CARDIO

EXERCISE	TIME	DISTANCE	REST

WHAT CHALLENGES DID YOU FACE TODAY?

HOW WILL YOU OVERCOME THESE CHALLENGES?

NOTES / PRAYERS / GRATITUDE

Date: ___ / ___ / ___

WHY AM I WORKING OUT TODAY?

Behold, I am coming soon, bringing my recompense with me, to repay everyone for what he has done. I am the Alpha and the Omega, the first and the last, the beginning and the end.
Revelation 22:12-13

TODAY'S WORKOUT GOALS:

EXERCISE	WT/Reps	WT/Reps	WT/Reps	WT/Reps	WT/Reps

CARDIO

EXERCISE	TIME	DISTANCE	REST

WHAT CHALLENGES DID YOU FACE TODAY?

HOW WILL YOU OVERCOME THESE CHALLENGES?

NOTES / PRAYERS / GRATITUDE

Date: ___ / ___ / ___

WHY AM I WORKING OUT TODAY?

You must serve only the Lord your God. If you do, I will bless you with food and water,
and I will protect you from illness.
Exodus 23:25

TODAY'S WORKOUT GOALS:

EXERCISE	WT/Reps	WT/Reps	WT/Reps	WT/Reps	WT/Reps

CARDIO

EXERCISE	TIME	DISTANCE	REST

WHAT CHALLENGES DID YOU FACE TODAY?

HOW WILL YOU OVERCOME THESE CHALLENGES?

NOTES / PRAYERS / GRATITUDE

WHY AM I WORKING OUT TODAY?

I will never forget your commandments, for you have used them to restore my joy and health.
Psalm 119:93

TODAY'S WORKOUT GOALS:

EXERCISE	WT/Reps	WT/Reps	WT/Reps	WT/Reps	WT/Reps

CARDIO

EXERCISE	TIME	DISTANCE	REST

WHAT CHALLENGES DID YOU FACE TODAY?

HOW WILL YOU OVERCOME THESE CHALLENGES?

NOTES / PRAYERS / GRATITUDE

WHY AM I WORKING OUT TODAY?

A cheerful heart does good like medicine, but a broken spirit makes one sick.
Proverbs 17:22

TODAY'S WORKOUT GOALS:

EXERCISE

	WT/Reps	WT/Reps	WT/Reps	WT/Reps	WT/Reps

CARDIO

EXERCISE	TIME	DISTANCE	REST

WHAT CHALLENGES DID YOU FACE TODAY?

HOW WILL YOU OVERCOME THESE CHALLENGES?

NOTES / PRAYERS / GRATITUDE

WHY AM I WORKING OUT TODAY?

As pressure and stress bear down on me, I find joy in your commands.
Psalm 119:143

TODAY'S WORKOUT GOALS:

EXERCISE

EXERCISE	WT/Reps	WT/Reps	WT/Reps	WT/Reps	WT/Reps

CARDIO

EXERCISE	TIME	DISTANCE	REST

WHAT CHALLENGES DID YOU FACE TODAY?

HOW WILL YOU OVERCOME THESE CHALLENGES?

NOTES / PRAYERS / GRATITUDE

WHY AM I WORKING OUT TODAY?

Anxiety in the heart of a man weighs it down, But a good word makes it glad.
Proverbs 12:25

TODAY'S WORKOUT GOALS:

EXERCISE	WT/Reps	WT/Reps	WT/Reps	WT/Reps	WT/Reps

CARDIO

EXERCISE	TIME	DISTANCE	REST

WHAT CHALLENGES DID YOU FACE TODAY?

HOW WILL YOU OVERCOME THESE CHALLENGES?

NOTES / PRAYERS / GRATITUDE

Date: ___ / ___ / ___

WHY AM I WORKING OUT TODAY?

For in Him we live and move and have our being
Acts 17:28

TODAY'S WORKOUT GOALS:

EXERCISE	WT/Reps	WT/Reps	WT/Reps	WT/Reps	WT/Reps

CARDIO

EXERCISE	TIME	DISTANCE	REST

WHAT CHALLENGES DID YOU FACE TODAY?

HOW WILL YOU OVERCOME THESE CHALLENGES?

NOTES / PRAYERS / GRATITUDE

Date: ___ / ___ / ___

WHY AM I WORKING OUT TODAY?

For the Spirit God gave us does not make us timid, but gives us power, love and self-discipline.
2 Timothy 1:7

TODAY'S WORKOUT GOALS:

EXERCISE

	WT/Reps	WT/Reps	WT/Reps	WT/Reps	WT/Reps

CARDIO

EXERCISE	TIME	DISTANCE	REST

WHAT CHALLENGES DID YOU FACE TODAY?

HOW WILL YOU OVERCOME THESE CHALLENGES?

NOTES / PRAYERS / GRATITUDE

Date: ___ / ___ / ___

WHY AM I WORKING OUT TODAY?

Therefore I tell you, whatever you ask for in prayer, believe that you have received it, and
it will be yours.
Mark 11:24

TODAY'S WORKOUT GOALS:

EXERCISE	WT/Reps	WT/Reps	WT/Reps	WT/Reps	WT/Reps

CARDIO

EXERCISE	TIME	DISTANCE	REST

WHAT CHALLENGES DID YOU FACE TODAY?

HOW WILL YOU OVERCOME THESE CHALLENGES?

NOTES / PRAYERS / GRATITUDE

Date: ___ / ___ / ___

WHY AM I WORKING OUT TODAY?

I pray that out of his glorious riches he may strengthen you with power through his Spirit in your inner being, so that Christ may dwell in your hearts through faith. And I pray that you, being rooted and established in love.
Ephesians 3:16-17

TODAY'S WORKOUT GOALS:

EXERCISE	WT/Reps	WT/Reps	WT/Reps	WT/Reps	WT/Reps

CARDIO

EXERCISE	TIME	DISTANCE	REST

WHAT CHALLENGES DID YOU FACE TODAY?

HOW WILL YOU OVERCOME THESE CHALLENGES?

NOTES / PRAYERS / GRATITUDE

WHY AM I WORKING OUT TODAY?

Now faith is confidence in what we hope for and assurance about what we do not see.
Hebrews 11:1

TODAY'S WORKOUT GOALS:

EXERCISE	WT/Reps	WT/Reps	WT/Reps	WT/Reps	WT/Reps

CARDIO

EXERCISE	TIME	DISTANCE	REST

WHAT CHALLENGES DID YOU FACE TODAY?

HOW WILL YOU OVERCOME THESE CHALLENGES?

NOTES / PRAYERS / GRATITUDE

Date: ___ / ___ / ___

WHY AM I WORKING OUT TODAY?

For we live by faith, not by sight.
2 Corinthians 5:7

TODAY'S WORKOUT GOALS:

EXERCISE	WT/Reps	WT/Reps	WT/Reps	WT/Reps	WT/Reps

CARDIO

EXERCISE	TIME	DISTANCE	REST

WHAT CHALLENGES DID YOU FACE TODAY?

HOW WILL YOU OVERCOME THESE CHALLENGES?

NOTES / PRAYERS / GRATITUDE

Date: ___ / ___ / ___

WHY AM I WORKING OUT TODAY?

May the God of hope fill you with all joy and peace as you trust in him, so that you may
overflow with hope by the power of the Holy Spirit.
Romans 15:13

TODAY'S WORKOUT GOALS:

EXERCISE	WT/Reps	WT/Reps	WT/Reps	WT/Reps	WT/Reps

CARDIO

EXERCISE	TIME	DISTANCE	REST

WHAT CHALLENGES DID YOU FACE TODAY?

HOW WILL YOU OVERCOME THESE CHALLENGES?

NOTES / PRAYERS / GRATITUDE

Date: ___ / ___ / ___

WHY AM I WORKING OUT TODAY?

But when you ask, you must believe and not doubt, because the one who doubts is like a
wave of the sea, blown and tossed by the wind.
James 1:6

TODAY'S WORKOUT GOALS:

EXERCISE

EXERCISE	WT/Reps	WT/Reps	WT/Reps	WT/Reps	WT/Reps

CARDIO

EXERCISE	TIME	DISTANCE	REST

WHAT CHALLENGES DID YOU FACE TODAY?

HOW WILL YOU OVERCOME THESE CHALLENGES?

NOTES / PRAYERS / GRATITUDE

Date: ____ / ____ / ____

WHY AM I WORKING OUT TODAY?

Then Jesus said, "Did I not tell you that if you believe, you will see the glory of God?"
John 11:40

TODAY'S WORKOUT GOALS:

EXERCISE	WT / Reps	WT / Reps	WT / Reps	WT / Reps	WT / Reps

CARDIO

EXERCISE	TIME	DISTANCE	REST

WHAT CHALLENGES DID YOU FACE TODAY?

HOW WILL YOU OVERCOME THESE CHALLENGES?

NOTES / PRAYERS / GRATITUDE

THANK YOU!

Thank you for supporting us at Zion Publishing! We pray this was a blessing to you!

For more books and journals, please visit our store page on Amazon and search for Zion Publishing or type this url in your browser:
https://www.amazon.com/stores/Zion-Publishing/author/B0CPTMTCTZ

You may also contact us at hello.zion.publishing@gmail.com.

We also have a community group to better support you along your journey! Join our Facebook group @ https://www.facebook.com/groups/1437898353466412

God bless!